Published By Adam Gilbin

@ Friedrich Kunze

Crockpot: Meal Plan for the Newly Diagnosed
Simple

Slow Cooker,meals,crockpot,crockpot Recipes

All Right RESERVED

ISBN 978-1-990666-72-8

TABLE OF CONTENTS

Crock Pot Keto English Muffin

INGREDIENTS:

- Ocean salt 1 pinch

- Baking soda 1/2 teaspoons

- Salt (as desired)

- Almond flour 3 tablespoons

- Coconut flour 1/2 tablespoon

- Spread (or coconut oil) 1 tablespoon

- Egg 1 large

Directions:

1. Take a medium-sized skillet, liquefy the margarine. It takes typically 20-30 seconds.
2. Pour coconut and almond flour, egg, salt into the softened spread and mix all that well.

3. Take the skillet from the hotness and add baking soda.
4. Open the Crock Pot, shower the lower part of the Crock Pot with cooking splash. Pour the mixture.
5. Cover the top and put on LOW for 2 hours. Really look at the status with a fork.
6. Remove the prepared «muffin» from the Crock Pot and eat with bacon cuts, cheddar or other breakfast staples.
7. Bon Appetite!

Scrambled Eggs With Smoked Salmon

INGREDIENTS:

- Salt and dark pepper freely

- Butter 2 tablespoon

- New chives voluntarily

- Smoked salmon ¼ lb(s)

- Eggs 12 pcs

- Weighty cream ½ cup

- Almond flour ¼ cup

Directions:

1. Cut the cuts of salmon. Put away for garnish.
2. Chop the remainder of salmon into little pieces.
3. Take a medium bowl, whisk the eggs and cream together.

4. Add a portion of the cleaved chives, season eggs with salt and pepper. Add flour.

5. Melt the margarine over medium hotness and fill the mixture

6. Spray within the Crock Pot with oil or cooking spray.

7. Add salmon parts of the combination, empty everything into the Crock Pot.

8. Cover the top and put on LOW for 2 hours.

9. Garnish the dish with staying salmon, chives.

10. Serve warm and enjoy!

Pork Stew With Oyster Mushrooms

INGREDIENTS:

- 1/3 cup full fat coconut milk preferably from a can

- 4 ½ tablespoons capers

- 1 large onion, peeled, chopped

- 3 pounds pork loin, cut into 1 inch cubes

- 1 teaspoon freshly cracked black pepper

- 3 tablespoons dried mustard

- 2 ¼ cups bone broth

- 3 pounds oyster mushrooms

- ½ cup ghee

- 3 tablespoons lard or coconut oil

- 2 cloves garlic, peeled, chopped

- 1 teaspoon Himalayan pink salt

- 3 tablespoons dried oregano

- ¾ teaspoon freshly ground nutmeg

- 3 tablespoons white wine vinegar

Directions:

1. Place a large heavy bottomed skillet over high heat. Add lard or coconut oil. When it melts, place pork in a single layer. Cook in batches if required. (If cooking in batches, add half the oil and place half the pork)

2. Cook until brown on all the sides.

3. Remove meat from the pan and place in a bowl.

4. Place the pan back over low heat. Add some more oil or lard if necessary. When the oil melts, add onion and garlic and sauté until onions are pink.

5.   Stir in oregano, ground nutmeg and mustard. Mix well. Add white wine vinegar and broth and mix well. Turn off the heat.
6.   Transfer into a crock-pot.
7.   Add the browned meat and the cooked juices. Mix well.
8.   Cover the crock-pot with the lid. Set the cooker on 'Low' and set the timer for 6 hours or on 'High' and set the timer for 4 hours.
9.   Stir in the mushrooms and 2 cups water. Cook on 'Low' and set the timer for 2 hours or on 'High' and set the timer for 1 hour.
10. Remove a little of the cooked gravy and add into a bowl. Add coconut milk and ghee and stir.
11. Pour it into the pot. Add capers and mix well.
12. Serve.

Luau Pork With Cauliflower Rice

INGREDIENTS:

- 3-4 teaspoons liquid smoke (optional)

- 2 ½ slices bacon, hickory smoked and nitrate free

- 4 cloves garlic, minced

- 2 pounds pork roast, shoulder or butt, trimmed of fat if desired

- 1 tablespoon Hawaiian black lava sea salt or more to taste

For cauliflower rice:

- 1 ½ tablespoons chicken broth

- Pinch salt

- 2 cups cauliflower florets

- ¼ teaspoon garlic powder

Directions:

1. To make cauliflower mash: Add cauliflower into the Crock-pot. Pour 2-3 tablespoons water.

2. Cover the crock-pot with the lid. Set the cooker on 'High' and timer for 45 minutes or until tender. Transfer into a bowl. Drain excess water.

3. Cool the cauliflower florets for a while and transfer into the food processor bowl.

4. Add garlic, chicken broth and salt. Pulse until a rice like texture is formed. Transfer into a bowl and keep warm.

5. Place bacon slices at the bottom of the slow cooker. Scatter garlic over the bacon.

6. Make cuts all over the roast.

7. Sprinkle black lava sea salt all over the roast and rub using your fingers, the salt well into the roast.

8. Place roast in the crock-pot with the fat side facing down. Sprinkle liquid smoke all over the top of the roast.

9. Cover the crock-pot with the lid. Set the cooker on 'Low' and timer for 8-10 hours or on 'High' and set timer for 4 hours initially and on 'Low' and set timer for 1-½ hours.

10. When done, remove pork and place on your cutting board. When cool enough to handle, shred with a pair of forks.

11. Add pork back into the pot. Also, add bacon and stir.

12. Cover the crock-pot with the lid. Set the cooker on 'Low' and timer for 1 hour.

13. Divide the pork among individual serving plates. Divide and place cauliflower rice on the side.

14. Serve hot.

Keto Low Carb Chili Recipe - Crock Pot Or Instant Pot

INGREDIENTS:

- 2 1/2 lb Ground beef

- 1/2 large Onion (chopped)

- 8 cloves Garlic (minced)

- 2 15-oz can Diced tomatoes (with liquid)

- 1 6-oz can Tomato paste

- 1 4-oz can Green chiles (with liquid)

- 2 tbsp Worcestershire sauce

- 1/4 cup Chili powder

- 2 tbsp Cumin

- 1 tbsp Dried oregano

- 2 tsp Sea salt

- 1 tsp Black pepper

- 1 medium Bay leaf (optional)

DIRECTIONS:

1. In a skillet over medium-high heat, cook the chopped onion for 5-7 minutes, until translucent (or increase the time to about 20 minutes if you like them caramelized).
2. Add the garlic and cook for a minute or less, until fragrant.
3. Add the ground beef. Cook for 8-10 minutes, breaking apart with a spatula, until browned.
4. Transfer the ground beef mixture into a slow cooker. Add remaining ingredients, except bay leaf, and stir until combined.
5. Place the bay leaf into the middle, if using.
6. Cook for 6-8 hours on low or 3-4 hours on high. If you used a bay leaf, remove it before serving.

7. Select the "Sauté" setting on the pressure cooker (this part is done without the lid).

8. Add the chopped onion and cook for 5-7 minutes, until translucent (or increase the time to about 20 minutes if you like them caramelized).

9. Add the garlic and cook for a minute or less, until fragrant.

10. Add the ground beef. Cook for 8-10 minutes, breaking apart with a spatula, until browned.

11. Add remaining ingredients, except bay leaf, to the Instant Pot and stir until combined. (For the Instant Pot version, it is recommended to also add a cup of water or broth.) Place the bay leaf into the middle, if using.

12. Close the lid. Press "Keep Warm/Cancel" to stop the saute cycle.

13. Select the "Meat/Stew" setting (35 minutes) to start pressure cooking.

14. Wait for the natural release if you can, or turn the valve to "vent" for quick release if you're short on time.

15. If you used a bay leaf, remove it before serving.

Chuck Roast With Mustard Sauce

INGREDIENTS:

- 1 oz heavy cream

- 1 tbsp yellow mustard

- 3/4 lb chuck roast cut in 1—inch cubes

- 1/2 chopped celery stalk

Directions:

1. Put together the seasonings: 0125 tsp. garlic powder, 1/2 tsp salt, and 0113 diced onion mix them with the cream and mustard inside the crock-pot blend thoroughly.

2. Upload the chopped celery stalk and the chuck roast cubes inside the crock-pot mix.

3. Cowl and cook dinner for four hours on high.

Beef & Broccoli

INGREDIENTS:

- 1/2 head broccoli cut in 1-iuch pieces

- 1/2 red bell pepper cut in 1-inch pieces

- 1/3 cup liquid amines

- 1/2 cup beef broth

- 1 lb flank steak cut in 1 to 2-inch cubes

Directions:

1. Prepare the seasonings: 1 1/2 tbsp of chosen
2. Sweetener, 1/ 2 tbsp grated ginger, 1 1/2 minced garlic cloves and salt to taste.
3. Add heed broth, amines and the steak cubes in a crock—pot.
4. Add the seasonings Cook for 5 hauls on low.
5. Add the broccoli and bell pepper on top and Cook for another hour.

17

Basic Nutty Granola

INGREDIENTS:

- 1 cup raw walnuts

- 1½ teaspoons ground cinnamon

- ¼ cup erythritol

- 1 cup raw pecans

- 1 cup raw almonds

Directions:

1. Grease a large crockpot.
2. In the prepared crockpot, add all INGREDIENTS:and stir to combine.
3. Set the crockpot on Low and cook, covered, for about 1½ hours.
4. Uncover and transfer the granola onto a large baking sheet.
5. Set aside to cool completely.

6. This granola can be preserved in an airtight container.

Heart Healthy Granola

INGREDIENTS:

- ½ cup raw pecans, chopped roughly

- ½ cup raw hazelnuts, chopped roughly

- ½ cup raw walnuts, chopped roughly

- ½ cup raw almonds, chopped roughly

- 1 teaspoon ground cinnamon

- 1/3 cup unsalted butter

- 1 teaspoon liquid stevia

- 1 teaspoon organic vanilla extract

- 1½ cups pumpkin seeds

- 1½ cups sunflower seeds

Directions:

1. Set a crockpot on High. Add butter and melt it.
2. Add liquid stevia and vanilla extract and stir to combine.
3. Add remaining INGREDIENTS: and stir to combine.
4. Cook, covered, for about 2 hours, stirring after every 30 minutes.
5. Uncover and transfer the granola onto large baking sheets.
6. Set aside to cool completely.
7. This granola can be preserved in an airtight container.

Egg Casserole With Sausage And Cheese

INGREDIENTS:

- 12 3/4 tablespoons grated cheddar cheese

- 1 green pepper, diced

- 9.6 oz. breakfast sausage links

- 9 1/2 tablespoons cottage cheese, rinsed and drained 1 1/4 teaspoons, divided

- 5-6 eggs, beaten until well-combined Black pepper, fresh ground

- 1 teaspoons Spike Seasoning

- 3 1/4 tablespoons sliced green onions 2 1/2 teaspoons onions for garnish

Directions:

1. Grease a crockpot with non-stick spray or olive oil. Then place cottage cheese into a fine

mesh colander. Put the cheese in the sink and rinse with water to wash away the creamy part.

2. In a frying pan, heat a teaspoon of olive oil over medium high heat and cook half of the sausage links until fully browned. Transfer the sausage onto a cutting board to cool down.

3. Now heat a teaspoon of oil and cool the remaining half of the sausage and move it to the cutting board too. You can cook the sausages together if your pan can accommodate them.

4. Heat a teaspoon of oil and brown the pepper pieces for about 2 or 3 minutes. You can cook them directly if you want them somehow crunchy.

5. Once done, cut the sausage links into halves and layer them in the crockpot along with diced or stripped green peppers.

6. Season with cottage cheese and then with the grated cheddar cheese. Top the mixture with sliced onions and top with black pepper and spike seasoning.

7. At this point, beat the eggs until well incorporated and then pour over the cut sausages, cheese and cottage cheese. Distribute the peppers and sausages in the cooking pot using a fork.

8. Close the lid in place and cook the mixture on low heat for 2 hours or more until the cheese is well melted and the eggs are firm in the center.

9. Finally, top with sliced green onions and enjoy the breakfast hot!

Turkey Crusted Crockpot Breakfast

INGREDIENTS:

- 1/2 chopped red bell pepper 1/4 chopped onion

- 1/4 teaspoons Mrs. Dash 1/4 teaspoons fennel seed 1/4 teaspoons sage

- 1/4 teaspoons onion powder

- 1/4 teaspoons garlic powder

- 0.5 pound lean ground turkey

- 12 tablespoons shredded Monterey Jack cheese 1/4 teaspoons pepper

- 1/2 cup cottage cheese

- 3 eggs

Directions:

1. Put the raw turkey meat in the slow cooker and then stir in onion, garlic, fennel, sage and the Dash. Stir the INGREDIENTS: together to blend.
2. Spread the turkey meat over the bottom of the slow cooker using the back of the spoon.
3. Then chop the veggies and now layer them over the poultry meat. In a medium-sized bowl, whisk the eggs.
4. Then stir in cottage cheese, pepper and salt into the whisked eggs and pour the cheese mixture over the veggies and turkey in the slow cooker.
5. Top the INGREDIENTS:with shredded cheese and cook them on low until set, preferably overnight. If you like it, use low fat turkey sausage as the crust.

Crock Pot Keto English Muffin

INGREDIENTS:

- Egg 1 large

- Sea salt1 pinch

- Baking soda1/2 teaspoons

- Salt (as desired)

- Almond flour3 tablespoons

- Coconut flour1/2 tablespoon

- Butter (or coconut oil)1 tablespoon

Directions:

1. Take a medium-sized skillet, melt the butter. It takes usually 20-30 seconds.

2. Pour coconut and almond flour, egg, salt into the melted butter and stir everything well.

3. Take the skillet from the heat and add baking soda.

4. Open the Crock Pot, spray the bottom of the Crock Pot with cooking spray. Pour the mixture.

5. Cover the lid and put on LOW for 2 hours. Check the readiness with a fork.

6. Remove the baked «muffin» from the Crock Pot and eat with bacon slices, cheese or other breakfast staples.

Bon Appetite!

Scrambled Eggs With Smoked Salmon

INGREDIENTS:

- Salt and black pepper at will

- Butter2 tablespoon

- Fresh chives at will

- Smoked salmon¼ lb(s)

- Eggs12 pcs

- Heavy cream½ cup

- Almond flour¼ cup

Directions:

1. Cut the slices of salmon. Set aside for garnish.
2. Chop the rest of salmon into small pieces.
3. Take a medium bowl, whisk the eggs and cream together.

4. Add a half of the chopped chives, season eggs with salt and pepper. Add flour.
5. Melt the butter over medium heat and pour into the mixture
6. Spray the inside of the Crock Pot with oil or cooking spray.
7. Add salmon pieces to the mixture, pour everything into the Crock Pot.
8. Cover the lid and put on LOW for 2 hours.
9. Garnish the dish with remaining salmon, chives.
10. Serve warm and enjoy!

Slow Cook Chicken Enchilada Soup Recipe

Ingredients:

- ½ cup chicken broth

- ½ cup chopped onion

- ½ cup diced bell pepper

- 1 can black beans, drained and rinsed

- 1 can diced tomatoes and jalapenos

- 1 can Enchilada sauce

- 1 cup shredded Monterrey Jack Cheese

- 1 pkg frozen corn

- 2 cups milk

- 2 whole chicken breasts

- 3 tbsp butter

31

- 3 tbsp flour

Directions:

1. In a saucepan, melt the butter over medium low flame. Add in the flour, continue stirring until bubbly and smooth.

2. Remove from heat and put the chicken broth and milk, slowly at a time, stir to keep it smooth.

3. Place the saucepan on the fire to heat again. Allow it to oil. Stir constantly until it thickens in a huge bowl, mix together the chicken broth and enchilada sauce.

4. Slowly whisk the rest of the milk until smooth. Put aside.

5. In a slow cooker, mix the beans, onion, bell pepper, tomatoes and corn.

6. Add the chicken breast on top of the mixture.

7. Add the sauce mixture on top of the ingredients in cooker.

8. Cover and cook for 6 to 8 hours on low or for 3 to 4 hours on high.

9. When it is time to serve, remove the chicken and shred and cut into bite size pieces.

10. Add the chicken back in the soup, combine together. Put cheese on top and serve.

Healthy Chicken And Dumplings Soup

INGREDIENTS:

- 6 dashes onion powder

- 4 (half a can) large flaky refrigerator biscuits

- 2 to 3 chicken breasts, thawed

- 1 can chicken broth.

- 2 cans cream of chicken soup

Directions:

1. Put the thawed chicken in the slow cooker. Top with chicken broth, diced onions and cream of chicken soup.
2. Cook on low for eight hours or high for four to six hours. Cook without stirring it.
3. Cut each uncooked biscuit into nine small pieces and add the chicken mixture. Cook on high for thirty minutes.

4. Take the chicken out from the Crock Pot and use fork to shred.

5. Return the chicken to slow cooker and then place everything in the pot. Serve hot.

Crock Pot Mexican Breakfast Casserole

INGREDIENTS: .

- 1 cup Chili fine powder

- 1 teaspoon Salt

- ¼ teaspoon Pepper

- ¼ teaspoon Eggs

- 10 Milk low fat

- Pork Sausage Roll - 12 ounces (I prefer Jones

- Dairy) Garlic powder - ½ teaspoon

- Coriander ½ teaspoon Cumin

- 1 teaspoon Salsa

- 1 cup Cheese (Pepper Jack if available) - 1 cup

- Toppings if required: Avocado salsa, sour cream, cilantroas per preference

Directions:

1. Put a skillet on low fire and cook pork wiener until it leaves its pink color.
2. Add every one of the flavors given and let it cool and set for some time.
3. Now take a medium bowl and whisk eggs and milk together.
4. Add the pork to the eggs and mix well so they get blended properly.
5. Take a stewing pot and oil its base and pour the combination you prepared.
6. Cook on high fire for 2 hours and 30 minutes.
7. You can put occasional fixings on it as per your taste.

Cauliflower Hash Browns Slow Breakfast Casserole

INGREDIENTS:

- Eggs - 12

- Milk - ½ cup

- Dry mustard - ½ teaspoon

- Kosher salt - 1 teaspoon

- Pepper - ½ teaspoon

- Cauliflower, shredded - 1 head

- Additional salt and pepper to season the layers as required Small onion, diced - 1

- Packaged pre-cooked breakfast sausages, sliced 5 ounces

- Shredded cheddar cheese 8 ounces

Directions:

1. First of all, oil a 6-quart slow cooker appropriately with cooking spray.
2. Mix well all the thing likes the eggs, milk, dry mustard, salt, and pepper.
3. From the destroyed cauliflower, take 33% part and layer it in the lower part of the sluggish simmering pot.
4. After that place 33% of the cut onion on top.
5. Use pepper and salt to prepare and finish off it with 33% piece of frankfurter and cheese.
6. Repeat a similar interaction by keeping two layers.
7. Pour the eggs combination over sluggish cooker
8. Cook on low for 5-7 hours and delay until eggs set appropriately and the top tone is browned.

9. Easy cooking tips: You can likewise cook the formula by utilizing moment pot cooker, which can diminish the cooking time impressively.

10. Actually look at the guidance of moment pot cooker, before using.

Brisket Chili

INGREDIENTS:

For the brisket:

- 2 tablespoons olive oil

- 1 clove garlic, peeled, finely chopped

- 1 small green bell pepper, discard seeds, finely chopped

- 1 tablespoon ground cumin

- 1 cup beef stock

- Salt to taste

- Freshly ground pepper to taste

- ¾ pound beef brisket, deboned

- 1 medium onion, peeled, finely chopped

- 4.5 ounces mushrooms, sliced

- 1 small jalapeño pepper, discard seeds, finely chopped

- ½ tablespoon chili powder

- ounces canned diced tomatoes

Directions:

1. Place a skillet over medium heat. Add 1-tablespoon olive oil. When the oil is heated, place the brisket in it.
2. Cook until brown from all the sides. Remove the brisket and place in the crock-pot.
3. Place the skillet back over heat. Add 1-tablespoon oil.
4. When the oil is heated, add onion, garlic, bell pepper, mushrooms and jalapeño pepper.
5. Sauté for 3-4 minutes. Stir in chili powder and cumin. Cook for a minute or two.
6. Turn off the heat. Transfer into the crock-pot. Pour broth all over the meat and vegetables.

7. Sprinkle tomatoes over the meat and vegetables.

8. Cover the crock-pot with the lid. Set the cooker on 'Low' and set the timer for 5 hours or on 'High' and set timer for 2 ½ hours. Turn the brisket every hour.

9. When done, remove brisket and place on your cutting board. When cool enough to handle, shred with a pair of forks.

10. Add meat back into the crock-pot. Stir well.

11. Cover the crock-pot with the lid. Set the cooker on 'Low' and set the timer for 1 hour.

12. Sprinkle salt and pepper and serve with mashed cauliflower or cauliflower rice.

Keto Crock-Pot Beef & Broccoli

INGREDIENTS:

- 1 cup liquid aminos

- 4 ½ tablespoons stevia or any other keto friendly sugar substitute of your choice

- 5 cloves garlic, minced

- 1 teaspoon salt

- 1 large red bell pepper, chopped into 1 inch squares

- 3 pounds flank steak, sliced into 1-2 inch chunks

- 1 ½ cups beef broth

- 1 ½ teaspoons ginger, freshly grated

- ½ -1 teaspoon red pepper flakes

- 2 medium heads broccoli, cut into florets

- Sesame seeds to garnish

Directions:

1. Set the crock-pot to 'Low' setting and let the crock-pot preheat.
2. Add steak, beef broth, garlic, ginger, aminos, sweetener, salt and red pepper flakes into the crock-pot.
3. Cover the crock-pot with the lid. Set the cooker on 'Low' and timer for 5-6 hours or on 'High' and set timer for 2 ½ - 3 hours.
4. Sprinkle in the red bell pepper and broccoli on top. Cook on 'Low' for another hour or until the vegetables are crisp as well as tender.
5. Toss well. Garnish with sesame seeds and serve as it is or with cauliflower rice.

Italian Pulled Pork Ragu (Instant Pot, Slow Cooker, Stove)

INGREDIENTS:

- 18 oz pork tenderloin

- 1 teaspoon kosher salt

- Black pepper, to taste

- 1 tsp olive oil

- 5 cloves garlic, smashed with the side of a knife

- 1 28 oz can crushed tomatoes

- 1 small jar roasted red peppers, drained (7 oz jar)

- 2 sprigs fresh thyme

- 2 bay leaves

- 1 tbsp chopped fresh parsley, divided

DIRECTIONS:

1. Season pork with salt and pepper. Press saute button to warm, add oil and garlic and saute until golden brown, 1 to 1 1/2 minutes; remove with a slotted spoon. Add pork and brown about 2 minutes on each side. Add the remaining INGREDIENTS:and garlic, reserving half of the parsley. Cook high pressure 45 minutes. Natural release, remove bay leaves, shred the pork with 2 forks and top with remaining parsley. Serve over your favorite pasta.

2. Season pork with salt and pepper. Heat a medium skillet over medium-high heat, add oil and garlic and saute until golden brown, 1 to 1 1/2 minutes; remove with a slotted spoon. Add pork and brown about 2 minutes on each side then transfer to the slow cooker with the garlic and the remaining

INGREDIENTS:, reserving half of the parsley. Cook 8 hours low. Remove bay leaves, shred the pork with 2 forks and top with remaining parsley. Serve over your favorite pasta.

3. Season pork with salt and pepper. Heat a large pot or Dutch oven over medium-high heat, add oil and garlic and saute until golden brown, 1 to 1 1/2 minutes; remove with a slotted spoon. Add pork and brown about 2 minutes on each side. Add the remaining ingredients to the pot including the garlic, reserving half of the parsley. Bring to a boil, cook covered on low until the pork is tender, and shreds easily, about 2 hours. Remove bay leaves, shred the pork with 2 forks and top with remaining parsley. Serve over your favorite pasta.

Slow Cooker Creamy Sausage And Broccoli Cheese Soup

INGREDIENTS:

- 8 oz velveeta, cubed

- 2 cups beef stock

- 2 tbsp garlic powder

- 1 cup cheddar cheese, shredded sharp

- 8 oz breakfast sausage, browned and crumbled

- 2 cups broccoli florets

- 1 cup diced carrots

DIRECTIONS:

1. In a large slow cooker, add sausage, broccoli, carrots, velveeta, beef stock, and garlic powder.

2. Cook on low 2-3 hours.

3. When soup is melted and creamy, add cheddar cheese.

4. Top with fresh cracked pepper and serve immediately.

Short Ribs With Creamy Mushroom Sauce

INGREDIENTS:

- 1/2 1]) beef short ribs, browned

- oz softened cream cheese

- 1/8 cup beef broth

- 1/2 cup white mushrooms

Directions:

1. Prepare seasonings: 1/4 tsp garlic powder, 1/4
2. tsp salt, and 1/ 4 tsp pepper.
3. Add seasonings to beef broth, cream cheese and mushrooms in a crock-pot. Put the short ribs on top.
4. Cover and cook on low for 6 hours. Mix every hour.

Beef Stroganoff

INGREDIENTS:

- 1 slice diced streaky bacon

- 1 tbsp tomato paste

- 1/2 cup beef stock

- 3 oz quartered mushrooms

- 6 oz beef in 1-iuch cubes

Directions:

1. Prepare seasonings: 1/ 3 sliced brown onions,
2. 2/ 3 crushed garlic clove, 1/3 tsp paprika
3. Add the seasonings to all the listed INGREDIENTS: in a crock-pot
4. Cover and cook on high for 6 bolus.

Fluffy Omelet

INGREDIENTS:

- 1 medium red bell pepper, seeded and sliced thinly

- 1 cup broccoli florets

- 1 small yellow onion, chopped

- 2 tablespoons fresh parsley, chopped

- ½ cup unsweetened almond milk

- 6 organic eggs

- 1/8 teaspoon red chili powder

- 1/8 teaspoon garlic powder

- Salt and freshly ground black pepper, to taste

Directions:

1. In a bowl, add almond milk, eggs, chili powder, garlic powder, salt and black pepper and beat until well combined.
2. Lightly grease a crockpot.
3. In the bottom of the crockpot, mix together the bell pepper, broccoli, and onion.
4. Pour egg mixture on top and gently stir to combine.
5. Set the crockpot on High and cook, covered, for about 1½-2 hours or until desired doneness of eggs.
6. Transfer the omelet onto a serving plate.
7. Carefully cut into 4 equal sized wedges.
8. Serve hot, garnished with the parsley.

Veggie Combo Omelette

INGREDIENTS:

- ¾ cup zucchini, chopped

- ¼ cup green bell pepper, seeded and chopped

- ¼ cup red bell pepper, seeded and chopped

- ½ cup Parmesan cheese, freshly grated

- 8 organic eggs

- 1 tablespoon olive oil

- 1 medium yellow onion, chopped

- ¾ cup carrot, peeled and chopped

- Salt and freshly ground black pepper, to taste

Directions:

1. In a large skillet, heat oil over medium heat and sauté onion for about 4-5 minutes.

2. Add remaining vegetables and cook for about 8-10 minutes.

3. Meanwhile, in a bowl, add cheese, eggs, and black pepper and beat until well combined.

4. Transfer the veggie mixture into a crockpot and top with egg mixture evenly.

5. Set the crockpot on High and cook, covered, for about 2 hours.

6. Transfer the omelet onto a serving plate.

7. Carefully cut into 6 equal sized wedges.

8. Serve hot.

Crock-Pot Veggie Omelet

INGREDIENTS:

- 1 cup feta cheese, crumbled

- 2 tablespoons of coconut oil

- Salt and pepper to taste

- 6 large eggs

- 4 cups spinach, fresh, chopped

- 1 ½ cups white mushrooms, sliced

- 2 cloves garlic, crushed

Directions:

1. Heat the coconut oil in Crock-Pot. Set aside. In a mixing bowl, combine garlic, eggs, salt, and pepper.
2. Add mushrooms and spinach to the mix.

3. Cover and cook for about 2 hours, or until omelet is set.
4. Check it at about 1 hour and 15 minutes into cooking time.
5. When the omelet is cooked, add the feta and fold in half. Transfer to serving plate.

Crock-Pot Breakfast Casserole

INGREDIENTS:

- 2 cups Monterrey Jack cheese, shredded

- 1 ½ cups spinach, fresh

- 1 ½ cups mushrooms, fresh, sliced

- 1 green bell pepper, diced

- 1 medium sweet yellow onion, diced

- 4 cups daikon radish hashed browns

- 1 lb. ground sausage, cooked, drained

- 12-ounce package bacon slices, crumbled, cooked, drained

- 1 dozen eggs

- 1 cup heavy white cream

- ½ cup feta cheese, chopped

- 1 teaspoon sea salt

- 1 teaspoon black pepper

Directions:

1. Place a layer of hashed browns on bottom of Crock-Pot. Follow with a layer of sausage and bacon, then add onions, spinach, green pepper, mushrooms and cheese.
2. In a mixing bowl, beat the eggs, cream, salt, and pepper together.
3. Pour over mixture in Crock-Pot. Cover and cook on LOW for 10-12 hours.

Breakfast Stuffed Peppers

INGREDIENTS:

- 1/4 cup almond milk

- 2 eggs

- 1 1/2 bell peppers, halved and seeded

- 1/4 cup finely chopped ham

- 6 tablespoons shredded cheddar cheese, divided

- 2 tablespoons chopped frozen spinach, thawed, squeezed dry 1 tablespoon chopped green onion

- Dash teaspoon salt

Directions:

1. Line a crockpot with tin foil then add the peppers and fill with the rest of the INGREDIENTS:.

2. Cook on low heat for about 3 to 4 hours or until eggs are cooked through.

Overnight Breakfast Casserole

INGREDIENTS:

- 1 red bell pepper, seeded and diced

- 0.4 pound rutabagas, peeled and shredded

- 3 1/4 tablespoons yellow onion, diced

- ounces bacon, chopped

- ounce bulk breakfast sausage, crumbled

- Softened ghee, to greasing the crockpot

- Green onions, for garnish

- Dash teaspoon cracked black pepper Dash
  teaspoon dry mustard
  1/2 teaspoon sea salt
  2 tablespoons full-fat coconut milk 3 1/4
  tablespoons almond milk

- 6-7 large eggs, beaten

  1 orange bell pepper, seeded and diced

Directions:

1. First grease the bottom and sides of a crockpot using softened ghee or palm shortening.

2. Then cook the onion, bacon and the sausage in the slow cooker until the onion is softened and the sausage browned, or for about 10 to 12 minutes.

3. Discard any excess fat. Now add in shredded rutabaga in the crockpot and press them down gently.

4. Add in the onion and meat mixture and bell peppers on top.

5. In a separate bowl, whisk together eggs, mustard, salt, milk and pepper. Pour into the crockpot.

6. Cook the mixture on low for 6 to 8 hours or until cooked through.

Crust Less Crock Pot Spinach Quiche

INGREDIENTS:

- Homemade sour cream1 cup

- Fresh chives2 tablespoons

- Sea salt1/2 teaspoon

- Ground black pepper1/4 teaspoon

- Ground almond flour1/2 cup

- Baking soda1/4 teaspoon

- Frozen spinach10 oz package

- Butter or ghee1 tablespoon

- Red bell pepper1 medium

- Cheddar cheese1 1/2 cups

- Eggs8 pcs

Directions:

1. Let the frozen spinach thaw and drain it well. Chop finely.

2. Wash the pepper and slice it. Remove the seeds.

3. Grade the cheddar cheese and set aside.

4. Chop the fresh chives finely.

5. Open the Crock Pot and spray the bottom and sides with cooking spray.

6. Take a little skillet, heat the butter over high heat on the stove, sauté the pepper until tender, for about 6 minutes.

7. In a large bowl combine together eggs, sour cream, salt and pepper.

8. Add grated cheese and chives and continue to mix.

9. In another medium-sized bowl, mix together almond flour with baking soda. Pour into the egg mixture, add peppers to the eggs mixture, pour gently into the Crock Pot.

10. Cover the lid and set on HIGH for 2 hours. Bon
    Appetite!

Crock Pot Brussels Sprouts Casserole

INGREDIENTS:

- Dried thyme½ teaspoon

- Garlic powder½ teaspoon

- Salt¼ teaspoon

- Pepper⅛ teaspoon

- Colby jack cheese1 cup shredded

- Brussels sprouts32 oz bag frozen

- Ground turkey sausage1 pound

- Eggs6 large

- Heavy cream2 tablespoons

Directions:

1. Open the Crock Pot and spray the bottom and sides with cooking spray.

2. Shred the cheese. Set aside.

3. Add about ⅔ of the bag of Brussels sprouts to the bottom of the Crock Pot.

4. In a medium-sized bowl whisk together eggs, heavy cream, thyme, garlic powder, salt and pepper.

5. Pour over the Brussels sprouts in the Crock Pot.

6. Take a medium-sized skillet, put over high heat, brown some sausage.

7. Add cooked sausage on top of eggs and the Brussels sprouts.

8. Top it all off with the remaining Brussels sprouts, add shredded cheese.

9. Cover the lid and cook on HIGH for 2 hours.

10. Bon Appetite!

Scrambled Eggs With Smoked Salmon

INGREDIENTS:

- Almond flour¼ cup

- Salt and black pepper at will

- Butter2 tablespoons

- Fresh chives at will

- Smoked salmon¼ lb(s)

- Eggs12 pcs fresh

- Heavy cream½ cup

Directions:

1. Cut the slices of salmon. Set aside for garnish.
2. Chop the rest of salmon into small pieces.
3. Take a medium bowl, whisk the eggs and cream together.

4. Add a half of the chopped chives, season eggs with salt and pepper. Add flour.

5. Melt the butter over medium heat and pour into the mixture

6. Spray the inside of the Crock Pot with oil or cooking spray.

7. Add salmon pieces to the mixture, pour everything into the Crock Pot.

8. Cover the lid and put on LOW for 2 hours.

9. Garnish the dish with remaining salmon, chives.

10. Serve warm and enjoy!

Garlic-Parmesan Asparagus Crock Pot

INGREDIENTS:

- Fresh asparagus12 ounces

- Parmesan cheese1/3 cup

- Pepper at will

- Olive oil extra virgin2 tablespoons

- Minced garlic2 teaspoons

- Egg 1 pcs fresh

- Garlic salt1/2 teaspoon

Directions:
1. Peel the garlic and mince it.
2. Wash the asparagus. Shred the Parmesan cheese.

3. Take a medium-sized bowl combine oil, garlic, cracked egg, and salt together. Whisk everything well.
4. Cover the green beans and coat them well.
5. Spread the cooking spray over the bottom of the Crock Pot, put the coated asparagus, season with the shredded cheese. Toss everything finely.
6. Cover and cook on HIGH for 1 hour.
7. Once the time is over you may also season with the rest of the cheese.
8. Bon Appetite!

Crock Pot Tomato Basil Soup

Ingredients:

- 4 left whole and peeled cloves garlic

- 10 basil leaves for garnish

- 3 28 Oz's cans whole peeled tomatoes

- For garnish, optional fresh grated Parmesan

- 1 qt chicken broth.

- 2 finely diced sweet onion, medium

- 1 tsp red pepper flakes, crushed

- 3 tbsp olive oil

- 3 finely diced and peeled large carrots

- 1 tbsp salt

Directions:

1. Place all the ingredients in a Crock Pot.

2. Cover and cook for five to seven hours on low until vegetables are soft and flavors are blended.

3. Let the soup cool down slightly.

4. Puree in batches in a blender until it becomes very smooth.

5. Serve immediately, or put the soup back in the crock pot and keep on low.

Tasty Black Bean Soup Recipes

Ingredients:

- 1 can Italian stewed tomatoes

- 3 can black beans

- 2 tablespoons taco sauce

- 1 1/2 cups vegetables chopped

- 2 cups vegetable or chicken broth

Directions:

1. Chop the vegetables using a blender or a food processor.
2. Add all the Italian stewed tomatoes and black beans without rinsing.
3. Add taco sauce and broth.
4. Mix with spoon.

5. Cook for eight to ten hours on low or five to six hours on high. The soup will taste better if you cook it longer.

Chicken Bacon Chowder

INGREDIENTS:

- ½ teaspoon garlic powder

- 1 small shallot, finely chopped

- 1 rib celery, chopped

- 1 small sweet onion, thinly sliced

- 1 cup chicken stock, divided

- 4 ounces cream cheese

- ½ pound bacon

- ½ teaspoon black pepper powder

- ½ teaspoon dried thyme

- ½ pound chicken breasts

- 2 cloves garlic, minced

- ½ small leek, cleaned, trimmed, sliced

- 3 ounces cremini mushrooms, sliced

- 2 tablespoons butter, divided

- ½ cup heavy cream

- ½ teaspoon sea salt

Directions:

1. Set the crockpot to 'Low' and preheat the crockpot.
2. Add garlic, leek, mushrooms, 1-tablespoon butter, sea salt, shallot, celery, onion, ½ cup chicken stock and black pepper powder into the crock-pot.
3. Cover the crock-pot with the lid. Set the cooker on 'Low' and timer for 1 hour.
4. Meanwhile, place a nonstick skillet over medium heat. Add 1-tablespoon butter. When butter melts, add chicken and cook until golden brown. Flip sides and cook the other

79

side until golden brown. It should not be cooked through only brown on the outside.

5. Remove chicken with a slotted spoon and place on your cutting board.

6. Pour remaining chicken stock into the skillet. Scrape the bottom of the pan to remove any browned bits that are stuck. Transfer the stock into the crock-pot.

7. Clean the skillet and place it back over medium heat.

8. Add bacon and cook until crisp. Remove bacon and place over paper towels. When cool enough to handle, crumble.

9. Stir in heavy cream, garlic powder, cream cheese and thyme into the crock-pot. Mix until it is free from lumps of the cream cheese.

10. Chop chicken into bite size cubes and add into the crock-pot. Also, add the bacon and mix well.

11. Cover the crock-pot with the lid. Set the cooker on 'Low' and timer for 6-7 hours.

12. Serve hot.

Greek Chicken

INGREDIENTS:

- ¼ teaspoon salt or to taste

- ½ jar marinated roasted red peppers, drained, diced (from a 12 ounces jar)

- ½ cup kalamata olives

- 1/3 cup chicken broth

- 1 tablespoon lemon juice

- ½ teaspoon dried thyme

- ½ teaspoon dried oregano

- A handful fresh basil, chopped

- 1 tablespoon olive oil or avocado oil

- 1 pound chicken thighs, skinless, boneless

- Black pepper powder or lemon pepper to taste

- ½ jar marinated artichoke hearts (from an 8 ounces jar), drained

- 1 small red onion, sliced

- 2 tablespoons red wine vinegar

- 1 tablespoon arrowroot starch mixed with 2 tablespoons water

- ¼ cup feta cheese, crumbled

- 2 cloves garlic, minced

Directions:

1. Place a skillet over medium high heat. Add oil and let it heat. Sprinkle salt and pepper over the chicken.

2. Add garlic into the skillet and sauté until fragrant. Place chicken and cook for 2 minutes each on both the sides.

3. Transfer into the crock-pot. Place artichoke hearts around the chicken and in the gaps between the chicken pieces.

4. Place onions on top. Add broth, lemon juice, vinegar, and herbs into a bowl and mix well.

5. Pour over the chicken.

6. Cover the crock-pot with the lid. Set the cooker on 'Low' and timer for 4 hours or set on 'High' and timer for 2 hours.

7. Add arrowroot starch mixture. Mix well. Cook for 10-15 minutes on or until thick.

8. Serve over cauliflower rice. Garnish with basil. Season with salt and pepper. Top with feta cheese and serve.

Slow-Cooker Stuffed Taco Peppers

Ingredients:

- 1 teaspoon garlic powder

- 1 teaspoon chili powder

- 1 ½ tablespoons olive oil

- 1 cup water

- 6 small red bell peppers

- 1 cup cauliflower rice

- 500 grams minced turkey

- 1 cup shredded Monterey jack cheese

Directions:

1. The first thing to do is cut off the stems on your peppers.

2. Scoop out the seeds on the inside, leaving a hollow shell.

3. In a bowl, mix together your minced turkey and spices.

4. Stir in the cauliflower and olive oil.

5. Mix in the Monterey jack cheese.

6. Scoop up some of the turkey mixture and pack it into each pepper shell.

7. Place them into a crockpot and pour a cup of water into the bottom.

8. Cook on high for 4 hours or low for 8. Top with a little extra cheese 10 minutes before they are done.

9. This makes a total of 6 servings of Crockpot Stuffed Taco Peppers.

Crock Pot Blueberry Lemon Custard Cake

Ingredients:

- 6 eggs separated

- 1/2 cup Coconut Flour

- 2 tsp lemon zest

- 1/3 cup lemon juice

- 1 tsp lemon liquid stevia

- 1/2 cup Swerve confectioners sweetener

- 1/2 tsp salt

- 2 cups heavy cream

- 1/2 cup fresh blueberries

Directions:

1. Place the egg whites into a stand mixer and whip until stiff peaks form. Set aside.

2. In another bowl, whisk the yolks and remaining ingredients together except blueberries.

3. Fold the egg whites a little at a time into the batter until just combined.

4. Grease the crock pot and pour the mixture into the pot.

5. Sprinkle the blueberries over the batter.

6. Cover and cook on low 3 hours or until a toothpick come out clean.

7. Allow to cool with cover off for 1 hour then place in the refrigerator to chill for 2 hours or overnight.

8. Serve cold with a little sugar free whipped cream if desired.

Self-Saucing Meatballs

INGREDIENTS:

- 1 egg

- 1/2 can chopped tomatoes

- 1/2 slice diced bacon

- 1/2 1]) ground beef

Directions:

1. Prepare the seasonings: 1/ 4 quartered onions and 1l2 chopped garlic.
2. Add seasonings to bacon in a food pmcessort Blend.
3. Add the ground beef and egg, and pulse until smooth.
4. Scoop 2 portion of the mixture and make into a meatball Place finished balls in a crock—pot.
5. Add the chopped tomatoes on top.
6. Cover and cook for 4 hours on high.

Braised Corned Beef Brisket

INGREDIENTS:

- 1/3 flat—cut corned beef brisket

- 1/3 tbsp browning sauce

- 1/3 tbsp vegetable oil

Directions:

1. Prepare seasonings: 1/3 sliced onion and 2
2. Sliced garlic cloves.
3. Apply a generous amount of browning sauce to both sides of the brisket
4. In a skillet, cook the brisket in preheated Vegetable oil for 5—8 minutes on both sides.
5. Place the brisket in a crock—pol. Scatter the Seasonings and add a tablespoon of water.
6. Cover and cook for 6 hours on low.

Summery Chicken Frittata

INGREDIENTS:

- 1 1/3 cups cooked chicken, chopped finely

- 1½ cups red bell pepper, seeded and chopped

- ¾ cup frozen chopped spinach, thawed and squeezed

- ¼ cup red onion, chopped

- 8 organic eggs

- Salt and freshly ground black pepper, to taste

Directions:

1. Grease a large crockpot.
2. In a bowl, add eggs, salt, and black pepper and beat well.
3. Place remaining INGREDIENTS: into prepared crockpot.

4. Place egg mixture over chicken mixture and gently stir to combine.
5. Set the crockpot on Low and cook, covered, for about 2-3 hours.
6. Cut into 8 equal sized wedges and serve.

Always-A-Hit Frittata

INGREDIENTS:

- 1 (14-ounce) can artichoke hearts, drained and chopped

- ¼ cup scallion, chopped

- 4 ounces feta cheese, crumbled

- 2 tablespoons fresh parsley, chopped

- 8 organic eggs

- Salt and freshly ground black pepper, to taste

- 1 (12-ounce) jar roasted red peppers, drained and chopped

Directions:

1. Grease a large crockpot.
2. In a bowl, add eggs, salt, and black pepper and beat well.

3. Place red peppers, artichoke hearts, and scallion into prepared crockpot.

4. Place egg mixture over vegetables and gently stir to combine. Top with cheese evenly.

5. Set the crockpot on Low and cook, covered, for about 2-3 hours.

6. Cut into 8 equal sized portions and serve warm, garnished with the parsley.

Crock Pot Mexican Breakfast Casserole

INGREDIENTS:

- 1/8 teaspoon coriander

- 1/8 teaspoon garlic powder

- ounces Jones Dairy Farm Pork Sausage Roll

- Avocado salsa, sour cream and cilantro: optional

- 1⁄4 cup Pepper Jack cheese 1⁄4 cup coconut milk
  4 eggs
  1⁄4 cup salsa

- Dash teaspoon pepper Dash teaspoon salt
  1/2 teaspoon chili powder 1/2 teaspoon cumin

Directions:

1. First cook the pork sausage in a large skillet over medium heat until it's no longer pink.

2. Season and add salsa then set aside to slightly cool down.

3. In a separate bowl, whisk the coconut milk with eggs then add in pork to the eggs.

4. Now add in Jack cheese and stir to blend. Grease the bottom of a slow cooker and pour in the egg mixture.

5. Finally cook on low for 5 hours or high for 2 1/2 hours. Serve topped with preferred toppings.

Cauliflower Breakfast Casserole

INGREDIENTS:

- 1 cup of shredded cheddar cheese

- 4 slices of low sodium, all natural turkey bacon, cooked and diced 1/2 small bell pepper, diced

- 1/2 small onion, diced

- Salt and pepper

- 1/2 head cauliflower

- 1/4 teaspoon pepper

- 1/2 teaspoon Himalayan salt

- 1/8 teaspoon dry mustard

- 2 tablespoons unsweetened almond milk

- 4 large eggs

Directions:

1. Coat a slow cooker with coconut oil or olive oil spray and set aside.

2. Then mix together dry mustard, eggs, salt, almond milk and pepper in a large bowl.

3. Put around 1/3 of the cauliflower in the bottom of the crockpot and top with one third of the bell pepper and onion.

4. Season with pepper and salt, and top with one third of the cheese and one third of the bacon. Repeat the layers two more rounds.

5. At this point, pour the egg mixture over the layers of the INGREDIENTS: in the crockpot.

6. Cook until the eggs are set and browned at the top, for about 5-7 hours or so. Serve and enjoy.

Crock Pot Turkish Breakfast Eggs

INGREDIENTS:

- Cherry tomatoes8 pcs

- Keto bread1 slice

- Eggs4 pcs

- Milk2 tablespoon

- Small bunch of parsley

- Natural yogurt at will4 tablespoon

- Pepper at will

- Olive oil1 tablespoon

- Onions2 pcs

- Red pepper1 pcs

- Red chili1 small

Directions:

1. Peel the onions and chop finely.
2. Wash parsley and chop finely. Wash the cherry tomatoes and dry with a paper towel.
3. Wash the pepper and chili, take off the seeds from the bell pepper and slice.
4. Cube the keto bread.
5. Spray the inside of the Crock Pot with oil or cooking spray.
6. In a large skillet, heat the oil, add the onions, pepper, and chili. Stir everything together.
7. Cook until the veggies begin to soften.
8. Put them in the Crock Pot and add the cherry tomatoes and bread, stir everything well.
9. Cover and cook on LOW for 4 hours.
10. Season with fresh parsley and yogurt.
11. Bon Appetite!

Bacon, Egg And Cheese Bread Boxes

INGREDIENTS:

- Bacon8 slices

- whole milk⅓ cup

- eggs12 large

- Hot sauce for dressing

- Keto bread1 loaf

- unsalted butter6 tablespoon

- American cheese8 slices

Directions:

1. Slice bacon into 1/2-inch pieces. Set aside.

2. Shred the cheese.

3. Remove about 1/4 inch of the crust from the ends of the keto loaf, cut the keto loaf crosswise into 4 pieces.

4. Using a fork make a box from each piece of keto bread.

5. Leave about 1/2-inch of bread around the bottom and walls.

6. Take a little skillet, melt the butter about 1 minute.

7. Brush the bread boxes inside and out with the melted butter, add salt.

8. Put small cheese slices at the bottom of keto bread box.

9. Open the Crock Pot and spread the cooking spray over the bottom and sides.

10. Place the boxes on the bottom of the Crock Pot.

11. Meanwhile, take a large bowl, whisk eggs and milk adding salt and pepper.

12. Add the mixture to the keto bread boxes, put the bacon slices over the top of the boxes.

13. Spread the shredded cheese.

14. Cover the lid and put on LOW for 3 hours.

15. Serve hot with hot sauce and additional salt and pepper.

16. Bon Appetite!

Persian Omelet Crock Pot

INGREDIENTS:

- Cilantro leaves¼ cup

- Parsley leaves¼ cup

- Fresh dill2 tablespoons

- Kosher salt and black pepper at will

- Pine nuts¼ cup

- Eggs9 large

- Whole milk¼ cup

- Greek yogurt at will1 cup

- Olive oil2 tablespoons

- Butter1 tablespoons

- Red onion1 large

- Green onions4 pcs

- Garlic2 cloves

- Spinach2 oz

- Fresh chives¼ cup

Directions:

1. Peel the onion cut thinly.
2. Chop carefully green onions. Chop chives.
3. Wash spinach after this carefully chops it.
4. Peel garlic and mince.
5. Finely cut cilantro and parsley, dill.
6. Take a saucepan melt the butter. Add red onion, stirring occasionally, it takes about 8-9 min.
7. Add green onions, garlic, continue cooking for 4 minutes.
8. Put the spinach, chives, parsley, cilantro, add salt and pepper at will. Remove the skillet, add the pine nuts.

9. Take a bowl, crack the eggs, add milk and a little pepper and whisk.

10. Mix the eggs with veggie mixture.

11. Open the Crock Pot and spread the cooking spray over the bottom and sides. Pour the mix into the Crock Pot.

12. Cover the lid and put on LOW for 3 hours. Serve with Greek yogurt.

13. Bon Appetite!

Broccoli And Cheese Stuffed Squash

INGREDIENTS:

- Italian season 1 teaspoons

- Mozzarella cheese1/2 cup

- Parmesan cheese 1/3 cup

- Cooking spray

- Salt and pepper at will

- Squash 1 pcs

- Broccoli florets2 cups

- Garlic 3 pcs

- Red pepper flakes1 teaspoons

Directions:

1. Wash and dry with a paper towel the squash. Cut in two halves. Take off the seeds. Set aside.
2. Wash broccoli thoroughly and cut into florets.
3. Peel garlic and mince it.
4. Spread the spray over the bottom and the sides of the Crock Pot. Put the halves in the Crock Pot.
5. Add a little bit water of room temperature to the bottom of the Crock Pot.
6. Cover the Crock Pot and put on LOW for about 2 hours, until squash is mild. Check the readiness once the time is over.
7. Take off the squash and let it cool for about 15 minutes.
8. Take a medium skillet, add pepper flakes and a little bit oil and cook for 20 seconds, stir it constantly.

9. Add broccoli, minced garlic to the skillet, continue to stir thoroughly, until the broccoli is tender.

10. Take the squash (previously cooled) and using a fork, take off the flesh of the squash. Add it to the medium bowl and conjoin with the broccoli mixture.

11. Shred carefully the Parmesan cheese, join salt and pepper at will, add seasoning to the mixture. Mix everything well and fill the squash.

12. Put the filled squash again in the Crock Pot, dress with mozzarella cheese each squash half.

13. Add a little bit water if needed to the bottom of the Crock Pot.

14. Cover and cook on LOW for about 1 hour.

15. Remove the dish and enjoy!

16. Bon Appetite!

Veggies And Chicken Minestrone Soup Crock Pot

Ingredients:

- 2 cans any kind of beans (drained)

- Vegetables (roasted broccoli,carrots,mushroom and asparagus left over)

- Salt and pepper to taste

- 1 can of tomatoes and its juice

- 1 can of corn and its juice

- 3 cups broth chicken (canned or fresh

Directions:

1. Add the drained beans in the Crock Pot.
2. Add the vegetables and juice from the tomato and corn.

3. Cover with chicken broth. If you are a
    vegetarian, you can opt for vegetable stock.
4. Cook for eight hours on low or 4 hours on
    high.

Crock Pot Baked Potato Soup

Ingredients:

- 8 cups chicken broth or stock

- 16 Oz's softened cream cheese

- For garnish shredded cheese, bacon

- 1 tbsp seasoned salt

- 1 diced, yellow onion, medium

- 10 minced garlic cloves

- 5 lbs russet potatoes, washed but unpeeled, diced into o. 5 in cubes.

Directions:

1. Add onion, seasoning, chicken stock, and potatoes to Crock Pot.
2. Cook six hours on high or ten hours on low.

3. Add the puree soup and softened cream cheese with an immersion blender until the cheese is well blended and about half the soup is combined.

4. Stir well, top with your favorite garnishes and enjoy.

Crock Pot Breakfast Casserole

INGREDIENTS:

- Fresh mushroom, sliced - 1 to ½ cups

- Fresh spinach - 1 to ½ cups

- Shredded cheese - 2 cups (Monterrey Jack preferred)

- Feta cheese, shredded - ½ cup

- Eggs - 1 dozen

- Heavy white cream - 1 cup

- Salt - 1 tablespoon

- Pepper - 1 tablespoon

- Brown jicama, hashed or brown daikon radish - 4 cups

- Cooked, crumbled, and drained bacon slices - 12 ounces

- Cooked, drained and grounded sausage - 1

- pound Onion, sweet yellow, chopped - 1

- Diced green bell pepper 1

Directions:

1. First of all, put a layer of hashed browns in the lower part of the cooker with low flame.
2. Then put the layer of bacon and hotdog over it.
3. Put every one of the flavors upon the layer.
4. Now take a bowl and whisk the eggs, cream, salt and pepper together.
5. Pour the combination of eggs in the cooker.
6. Cover it and let it cook for 6 hours on high fire or for 12 hours on low flame.

Keto Slow Cooker Bacon-Mushroom Breakfast

INGREDIENTS:

- Kale leaves large, shredded 8

- Nos. Ghee 1 Tablespoons.

- Parmesan cheese 1 Cup

- Avocado and green leaves (Optional)

- Bacon large, sliced 3½ Ounces

- White mushrooms, chopped 2½

- Ounces Eggs 6 Nos.

- Shallots, chopped 3 Tablespoons Bell pepper, chopped - ¾ Cup

Directions:

1. Clean the kale leaves, eliminate the hard stems and hack into little pieces.

2. In a skillet cook the bacon, till it becomes fresh and add mushrooms, red pepper, and shallot.
3. Add kale and cut down the fire and let the kale become delicate in the skillet.
4. Now take a medium bowl and beat all eggs, add pepper and salt.
5. In the stewing pot, add ghee and allow it to become hot. Spread the ghee on all side of the cooker.
6. Put the sautéed vegetable into the foundation of the cooker.
7. Spread the cheddar over the vegetables.
8. Then, add the beaten eggs on top.
9. Just mix it gently.
10. Set the cooker on low hotness and cook for around 6 hours.
11. Serve hot with cut avocado and green leaves.

Chocolate Chicken Mole

INGREDIENTS:

- ¼ teaspoon guajillpo chili powder

- Sea salt to taste

- Black pepper powder to taste

- 1 small onion, chopped

- 3 whole tomatoes, peeled, deseeded, chopped

- 2 tablespoons creamy almond butter

- ¼ teaspoon ground cinnamon powder

- ½ avocado, peeled, pitted, chopped

- 1 jalapeño, deseeded, chopped

- A handful fresh cilantro, chopped

- 1 pound chicken pieces bone-in, skinless

- 1 tablespoon ghee

- 2 cloves garlic, crushed or minced

- 3 dried New Mexico chili peppers, rehydrated, chopped

- 1 ¼ ounce keto friendly dark chocolate (70%)

- ½ teaspoon cumin powder

Directions:

1. Sprinkle salt and pepper over the chicken. Place a skillet with ghee over medium heat.
2. When ghee melts, add chicken and cook until brown on all the sides. Transfer into the crock-pot.
3. Place the skillet back over heat. Add onions and cook until soft.
4. Stir in the garlic and cook until fragrant. Transfer into the crock-pot.

5. Stir in the tomatoes, almond butter, chili peppers, dark chocolate, cumin powder, chili powder, pepper and cinnamon powder.

6. Cover the crock-pot with the lid. Set the cooker on 'Low' and timer for 4 hours or set on 'High' and timer for 2 hours.

7. Remove chicken with a slotted spoon and place on your cutting board.

8. Add chicken back into the pot and mix well.

9. Divide into plates. Place avocado, jalapeño and cilantro on top and serve.

Lamb Curry With Spinach

INGREDIENTS:

- 1 tablespoon fresh ginger, crushed

- 3 whole cloves

- ½ teaspoon turmeric powder

- ½ tablespoon garam masala powder

- 8.8 ounces lamb, cubed

- ounces canned tomatoes, chopped

- Salt to taste

- 1 clove garlic, crushed

- 1 teaspoon ground cardamom

- 1 teaspoon ground coriander

- ¼ teaspoon chili powder

- 1 teaspoon cumin powder

- ounces frozen spinach, thawed

- 1 small red onion, sliced

Directions:

1. Squeeze the spinach lightly of excess moisture.

2. Add garlic, cardamom, coriander, chili powder, cumin powder, spinach, onion, ginger, cloves, turmeric powder, garam masala powder, lamb, tomatoes and salt into the crock-pot and mix well.

3. Cover the crock-pot with the lid. Set the cooker on 'Low' and timer for 4-5 hours or set on 'High' and timer for 2- 2 ½ hours or until the meat is tender.

4. Mix well and serve.

Poached Salmon

INGREDIENTS:

- 2 cups dry white wine

- 2 shallots, thinly sliced

- 10-12 sprigs fresh herbs of your choice

- 2 teaspoons kosher salt

- Freshly ground pepper

- Salt to taste

- 4 cups water

- 2 lemons, thinly sliced

- 2 bay leaves

- 2 teaspoons whole black peppercorns

- 8 salmon fillets

Directions:

1. Add water, lemon, dry white wine, shallots, fresh herbs, salt and peppercorns into the crock-pot.

2. Cover the crock-pot with the lid. Set the crockpot on 'High' and set the timer for 30 minutes.

3. Sprinkle salt and pepper over the salmon and place in the crockpot.

4. Set on 'High' for 1 hour. Keep a check on the salmon after 45 minutes of cooking. Cook until done.

5. Remove with a slotted spoon and place on a serving platter.

6. Sprinkle coarse sea salt and drizzle oil and serve with lemon wedges.

Crock Pot Sugar Free Bbq Pulled Chicken

INGREDIENTS:

- 3 pounds boneless skinless chicken thighs

- 1 teaspoon smoked paprika

- 1 teaspoon onion powder

- 1 teaspoon cumin

- 1/2 teaspoon salt

- 1/4 teaspoon pepper

- 1/2 cup water

- 1/4 cup apple cider vinegar

- 1 cup sugar free ketchup use my recipe from cookbook if you have it

- 1 teaspoon maple extract

- 1/4 teaspoon cumin

- 1/4 teaspoon salt

- 1 tablespoon cocoa powder unsweetened

- 1/2 teaspoon clear liquid stevia

Directions:

1. Place the chicken on a baking sheet.
2. Whisk the paprika, onion powder, cumin, salt and pepper together.
3. Rub the dry seasonings onto the chicken on both sides. Set aside.
4. Pour the water, apple cider vinegar, and ketchup into the bottom of the crock pot.
5. Stir until combined then add the remaining INGREDIENTS:to the crock pot.
6. Stir well then add the chicken thighs to the crock pot.
7. Cover and cook on high 4 hours or low 8 hours.

8. Uncover when finished cooking and shred thighs with 2 forks.
9. Enjoy over coleslaw or in a low carb tortilla as a burrito.

Easy Crockpot Chicken Stew

INGREDIENTS:

- 2 cups chicken stock

- 2 medium carrots, peeled and finely diced

- 2 celery stalks, diced

- ½ onion, diced

- 28 oz skinless and deboned chicken thighs diced into 1" pieces

- 1 1 spring fresh rosemary or ½ teaspoon dried rosemary

- 3 garlic cloves, minced

- ¼ tsp dried thyme

- ½ tsp dried oregano

- 1 cup fresh spinach

- ½ cup heavy cream

- Salt and pepper, to taste

- Xantham gum, to desired thickness starting at ⅛ teaspoon

Directions:

1. Place the chicken stock, carrots, celery, onion, chicken thighs, rosemary, garlic, thyme, and oregano into a 3-quart crockpot or larger. Cook on high for 2 hours or on low for 4 hours.
2. Add salt and pepper, to taste.
3. Stir in spinach and the heavy cream.
4. Sprinkle and thicken with xantham gum to desired thickness starting at ⅛th teaspoon. Continue to whisk until mix and cook for another 10 minutes.

Italian Beef For Sandwiches

INGREDIENTS:

- 1/4 tsp dried parsley

- 1/4 tsp dried oregano

- 1/4 (51b) rump roast

- 1/4 bay leaf

- 1/4 (0.7oz) package dry Italian—style salad

- Dressing mix

Directions:

1. Prepare seasonings: 1/ 2 cup water with salt, Garlic powder and ground black pepper to taste.
2. Add the seasonings to the salad dressing mix
3. Add the bay leaf, parsley and oregano. It well

4. Put the mast in the crock-pot and pour the Resulting salad dressing mixture. Mix well

5. Cover and cook for 4 to 5 hours on high

London Broil

INGREDIENTS:

- 1/2 lb flank steak

- 1/4 package dry onion soup mix

- 1/4 can condensed cream of mushroom soup

- 1/4 can condensed tomato soup

Directions:

1. Place meat on a crock—pol. Slice it if necessary
2. To fit
3. Mix mushroom and tomato soup thoroughly
4. And pour this over the meal.
5. Emblazon with dry onion soup mix on the top'
6. Cover and cook for 8 bolus on low

Japanese Pumpkin Dip

Ingredients:

- Unsalted spread (or ghee) 2 tablespoons

- Weighty cream (or coconut cream) 2 cups

- Garlic powder 1 tablespoon

- Ocean salt 1 teaspoon new

- Rosemary 4 sprigs

- Water or broth 1/2 - 1 cup

- Pumpkin seeds 1/3 cup

- Japanese pumpkin 3 lbs

- Olive oil 1/4 cup

- Ocean salt 1 teaspoon

- White onion 1 medium

Directions:

1. Wash the Japanese pumpkin and eliminate the seeds.

2. Chop into 2-inch cubes.

3. Open the Crock Pot and splash the cooking shower over the bottom.

4. Put the 3D shapes onto the lower part of the Crock Pot, sprinkle with olive oil and season with salt.

5. Cover and put on HIGH for 2 hours.

6. Peel and slash finely the white onion, cook it until brilliant in a little pan with unsalted butter.

7. Once the onion is clear, put it into a bowl. Set aside.

8. Whip weighty cream in a food processor for around 5 minutes. 8. Add the cooked onion, garlic powder, salt and new rosemary. Mix everything well.

9. Once the pumpkin is prepared, let it cool a tad and strip the skin off.

10. Mix the stripped pumpkin in the food processor along with the whipped cream combination until creamy.
11. Transfer the pumpkin soup into the Crock Pot and put on LOW for 1 more hour.
12. Serve with pumpkin seeds!
13. Enjoy warm!

Blackberry Egg Keto Bake

Ingredients:

- Eggs 5 large margarine (melted) coconut flour

- Ground new ginger 1 tablespoon

- 3 tablespoons 1 teaspoon vanilla 1/4 teaspoon

- Fine ocean salt 1/3 teaspoon

- Zing of lime 1/2 tablespoon new

- Rosemary 1 teaspoon

- New blackberries 1/2 cup

Directions:

1. Open the Crock Pot and splash the cooking shower over the bottom.
2. Melt the spread in a little saucepan.
3. Finely hack new rosemary.
4. Place newly broke eggs, softened margarine, coconut flour, newly ground ginger, vanilla,

salt, zing into a blender and interaction for around two minutes on high.

5. The blend should be completely consolidated and smooth.

6. Add the rosemary and heartbeat for a couple of times until the rosemary is simply incorporated.

7. Put the egg combination into the Crock Pot, add the blackberries.

8. Cover the Crock Pot and set on HIGH for 60 minutes, until the egg combination puffs and is completely cooked through.

9. Let it cool for a couple of moments once cooked. Add cleaved rosemary.

10. Bon Appetite!

Slow Cooked Summer Vegetables

Ingredients:

- ½ cup mushrooms, sliced

- ½ cup grape tomatoes

- 1 ¼ cups zucchini, sliced

- ¼ cup olive oil

- ¼ cup balsamic vinegar

- ½ tablespoon fresh thyme, chopped

- 1 tablespoon fresh basil, chopped

- 1 cup okra, sliced

- ¾ cup red onion, chopped into chunks

- 1 cup yellow bell pepper, sliced

- Salt to taste

- Pepper to taste

Directions:

1. Add olive oil and vinegar into a bowl and whisk until well combined.
2. Add basil and thyme and stir.
3. Add okra, red onion, bell pepper, mushrooms, grape tomatoes and zucchini into the crock-pot and toss well.
4. Pour the oil mixture over it. Mix until the vegetables are well coated with the oil mixture.
5. Cover the crock-pot with the lid. Set the cooker on 'Low' and set timer for 3 hours or set on 'High' and timer for 1 ½ hours or until the vegetables are tender.
6. Stir after every 40-60 minutes. Season with salt and pepper.
7. Serve hot.

Crockpot Turkey Breast

Ingredients:

- 1 tablespoon arrowroot powder mixed with 2 tablespoons water

- 1 bone-in turkey breast (2.5-3 pounds) thawed, skinless

- 1 yellow onion, chopped into chunks

- ½ cup chicken broth

- 3 tablespoons butter

- 3 stalks celery, chopped

- 6-8 baby carrots

For seasonings:

- A large pinch dried parsley

- 1/8 teaspoon dried thyme

- ½ teaspoon seasoned salt

- ¼ teaspoon pepper powder

- ½ tablespoon dried minced garlic

- ½ teaspoon paprika

- ½ teaspoon Italian seasoning

- A large pinch dried sage

Directions:

1. Spray some cooking spray in the inside of the Instant Pot.

2. Spread celery at the base of the pot. Next place half the onion followed by carrots. Drizzle chicken broth over it.

3. Place turkey in the crock-pot over the vegetables with the breast side facing down. Place the remaining onion chunks and 2 tablespoons butter pieces inside the turkey at different places.

4. Mix together the seasonings in a bowl. Rub this mixture over the turkey. Add remaining butter into a small saucepan and let it melt. Brush it over the turkey.

5. Cover the crock-pot with the lid. Set the cooker on 'Low' and set timer for 5-7 hours or set on 'High' and timer for 3-4 hours or until the meat is very tender and the internal temperature of the turkey shows 165 degrees F with a cooking thermometer.
6. Remove turkey with a slotted spoon and place on your cutting board. When cool enough to handle, discard the bones. Cut the meat into slices and serve with gravy.
7. To make gravy: Let the liquid in the pot sit for a while; remove the fat that is floating on the top.
8. Cook on 'High' for a while, stirring constantly. Add arrowroot mixture and stir frequently until thick.
9. Taste and adjust the seasonings if necessary.